Marv's Healthy Choice

Written by Bigg Marv
with Cyrus Webb

Illustrated by C. A. Webb

Written by Bigg Marv with Cyrus Webb
Illustrated by C. A. Webb

Distributed by Conversations Media Group

Printed in the United States of America

Acknowledgements

From Bigg Marv: Thanks first to God for giving me gifts to share with the world. I want to say thanks to my grandmother and grandfather for helping raise me and teaching me to be the man that I am. Special thanks to my Great-Uncle Abraham, my cousin MC Hammer and his wife Stephanie as well as those who have been by my side since day one. I love and thank you all. And last but not least thanks to Cyrus Webb for helping me share this important message about a healthy lifestyle with the world.

From Cyrus Webb/C.A. Webb: Thanks to my Creator for endowing me with the ability to use my gifts each and every day. I thank my family for their continued support especially my nephew A'tavion and my cousin Jaila for allowing me to share my love of reading with them. To my supporters around the world I thank you for believing in my work. And to Bigg Marv: thanks for the opportunity to work with you on this project!

Marv's Healthy Choice

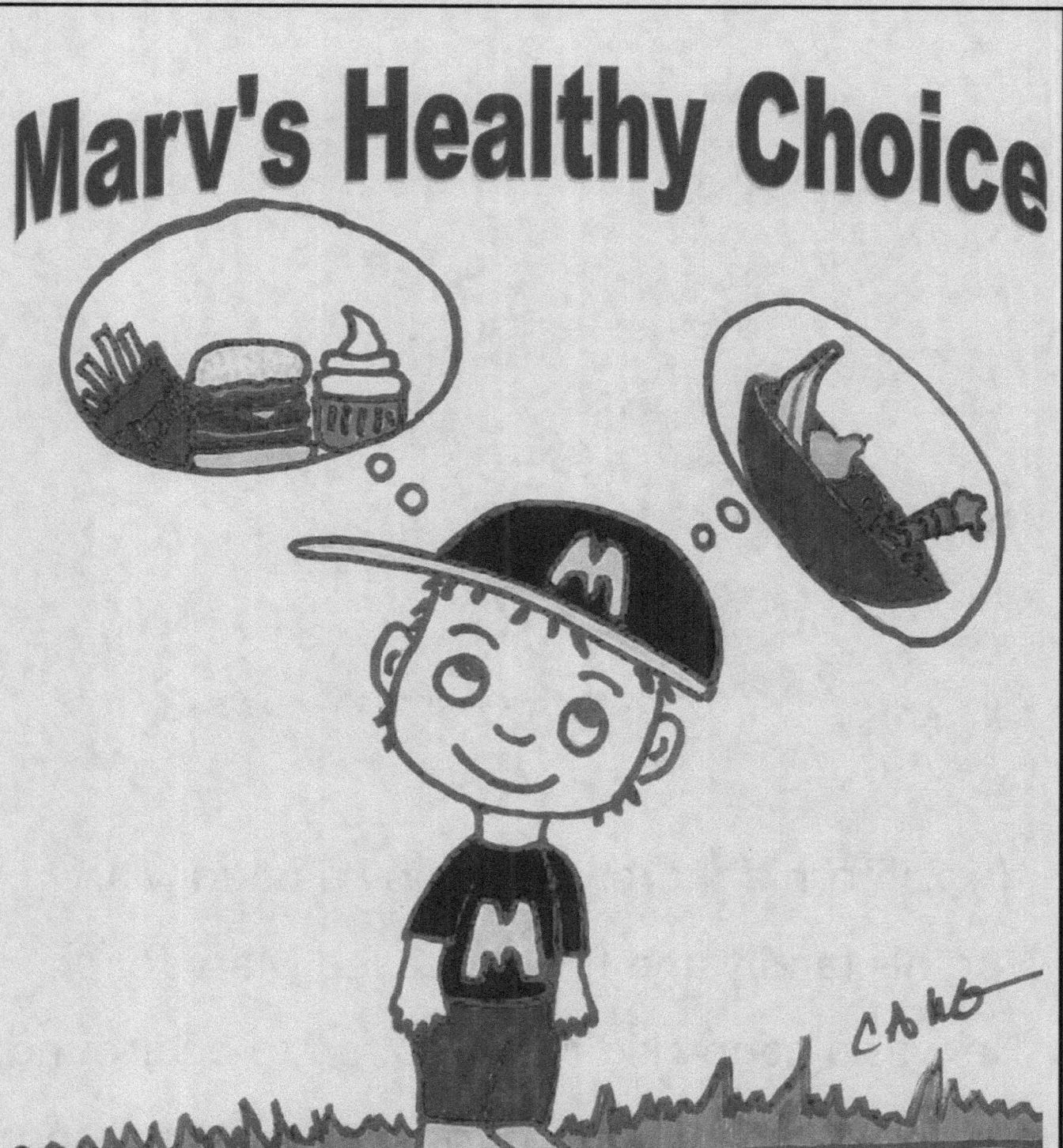

Written by Bigg Marv
with Cyrus Webb
Illustrated by C. A. Webb

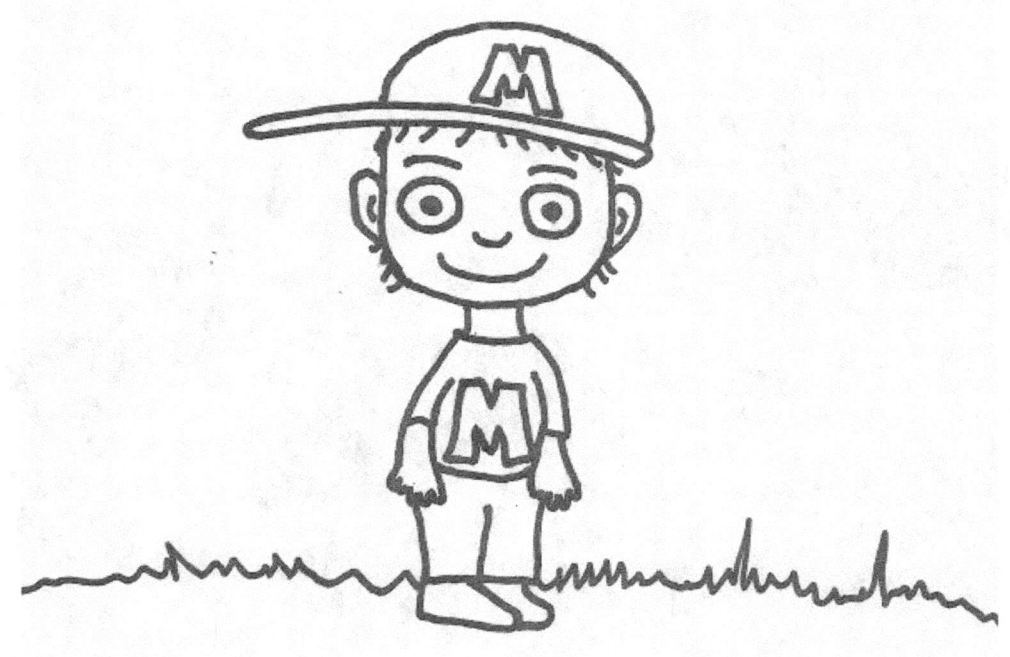

In California there lived a boy named Marvin,

Who his family and friends called Marv for short.

He was a happy kid that was fun to be around.

He enjoyed listening to music and watching sports

Marv could make you laugh when you were unhappy.

He cracked jokes, causing you to smile when you were feeling down.

When he was with you it was hard not to be upbeat.

Marv helped turn that frown upside down.

Though Marv was well liked and a good kid,

There was one thing he did that wasn't good.

He overdid it when eating sweets

And other kinds of unhealthy food.

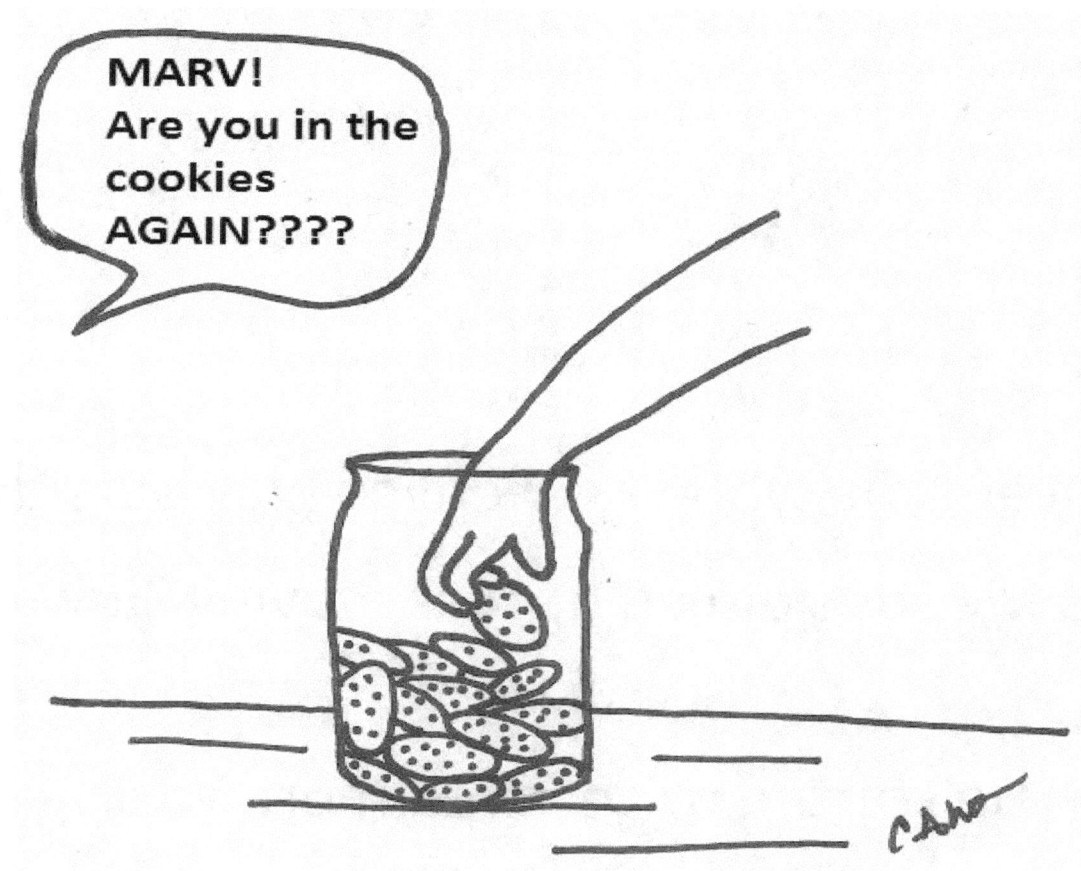

Marv would eat lots of cookies

And filled his lunchbox with them for snack.

When it came to his mom's fried chicken,

For seconds and thirds he would always go back!

Over time when he went to play outside

Marv's friends noticed he was moving slower than slow.

He started to get tired more easily,

And then he noticed his stomach began to grow!

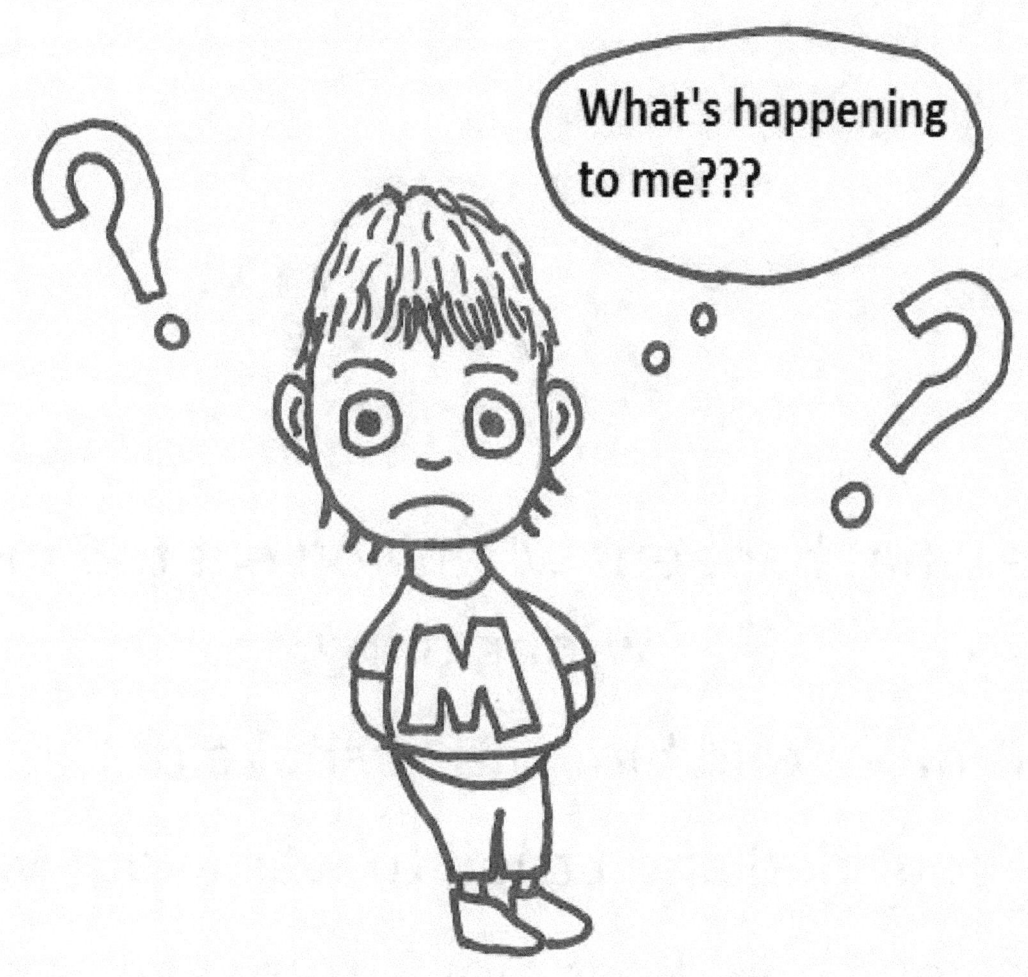

"What's happening to me?" Marv said one day when he couldn't get his clothes to fit right.

It seemed as though everything had shrunk,

Even his pants were way too tight!

"This is what happens when you eat too much of the wrong thing,"

His mom told him with a shake of the head.

"Your dad and I tried to warn you, Marv,

That you should eat more fruits and vegetables instead."

"Is that why I feel differently?"

Marv asked with sadness in his voice.

He didn't realize that looking and feeling better

Was something that was a choice.

"Don't be too hard on yourself son," his dad told him.

"When it comes to our diet we all make mistakes.

When you eat healthy and exercise,

Your body will stay in shape."

Marv knew he had to make a choice
To be the best person he could be.
He decided to start that very day
Watching what he chose to eat.

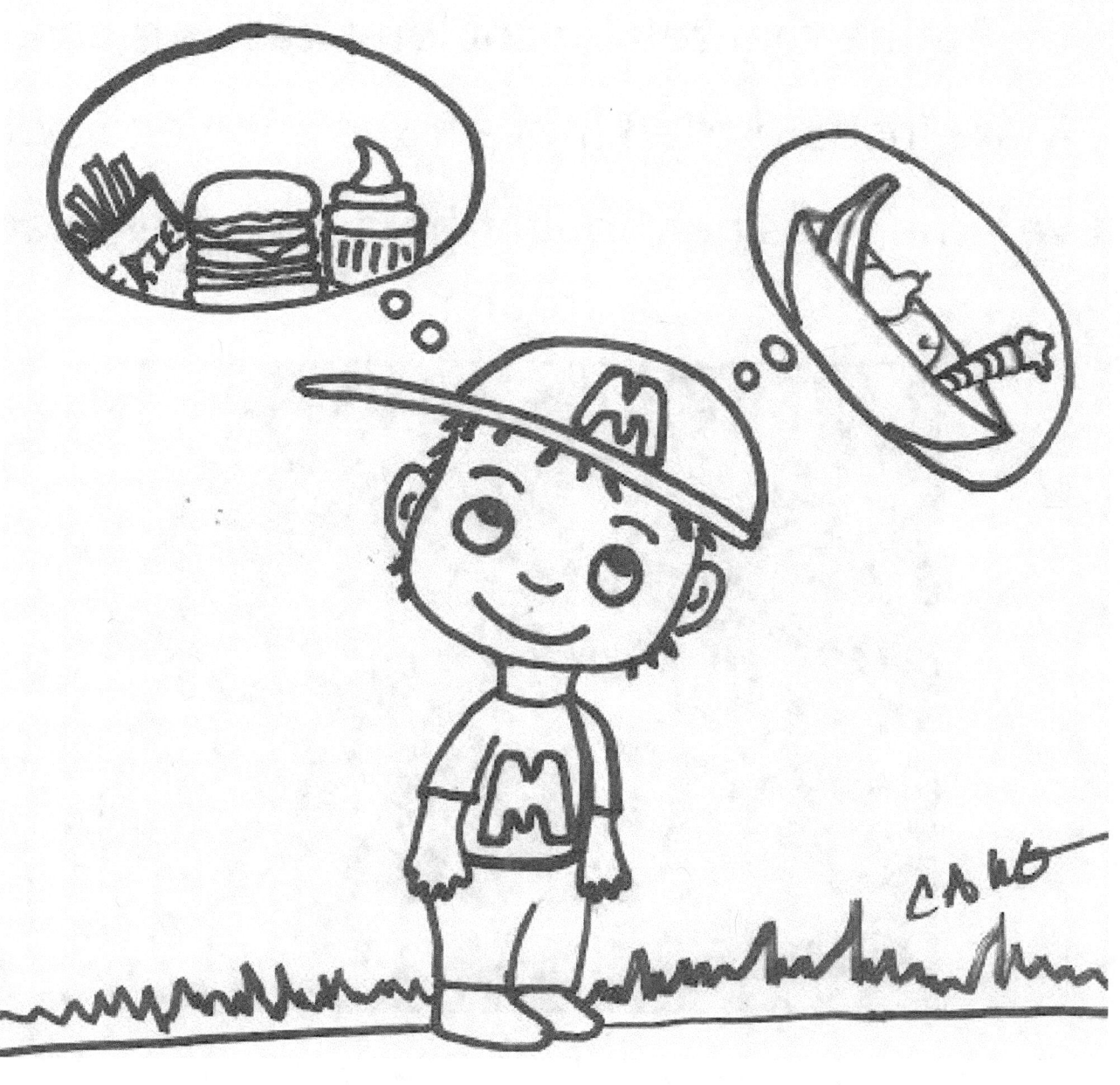

He still liked his mom's chicken,

But he realized he couldn't eat as much.

Marv instead tried more fruits and vegetables,

Even the ones he thought he didn't even want to touch.

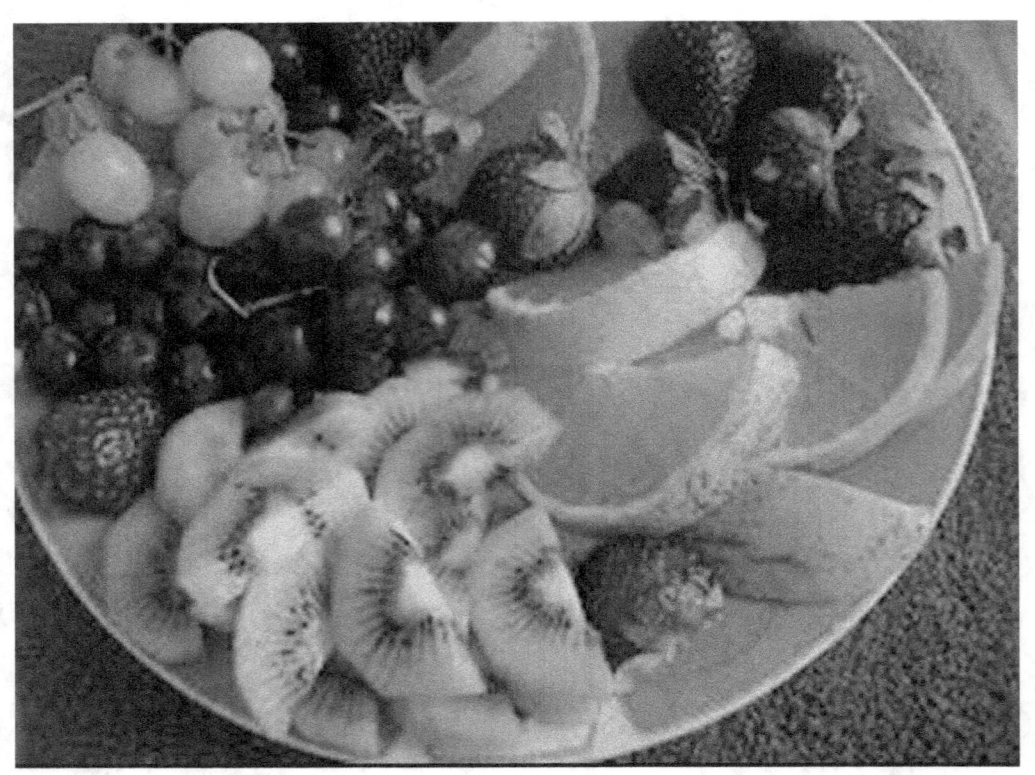

Instead of spending his time playing games inside the house,

Marv started spending more time with friends jogging and taking walks.

Together they made plans to be healthier

And along the way they laughed and talked.

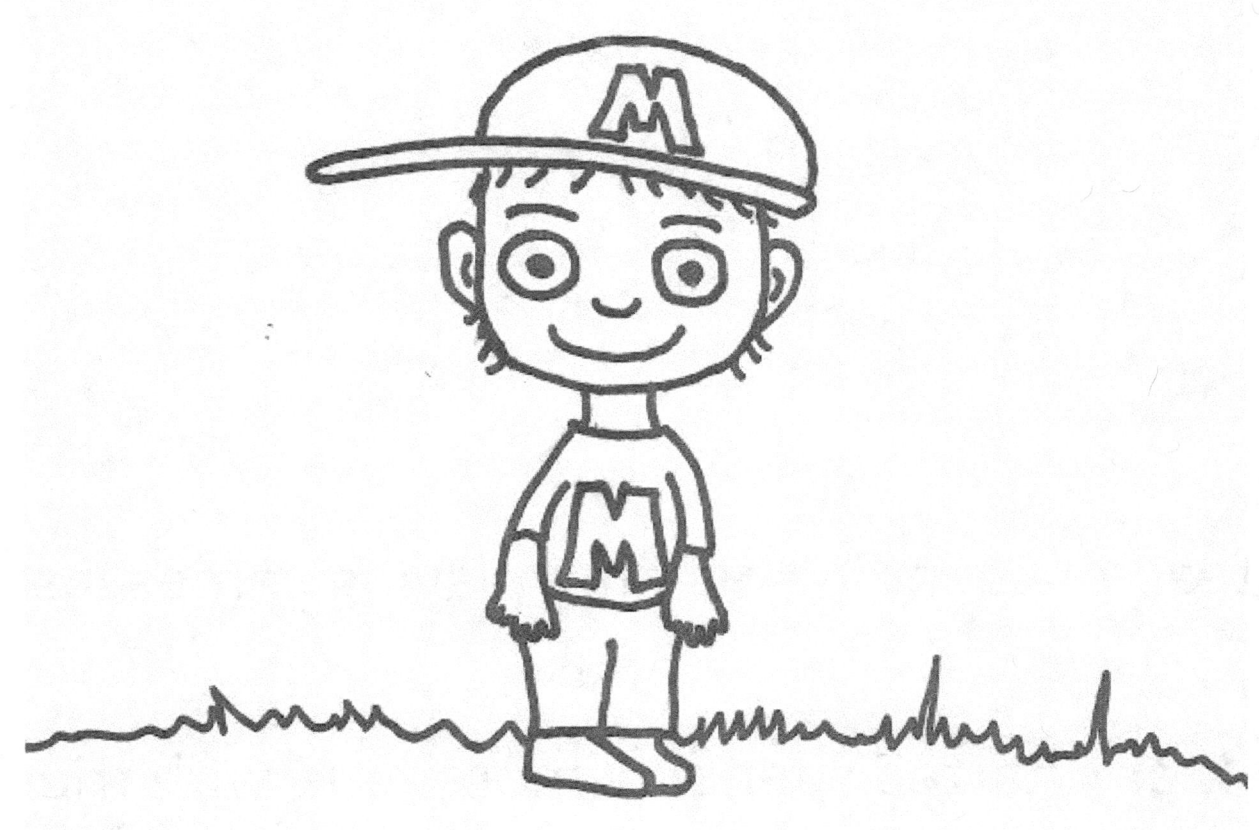

Before long Marv found his energy again,

And his clothes were fitting as they should.

Marv vowed to keep living and eating healthier

He wanted to show others that thought they couldn't do better, that they could.

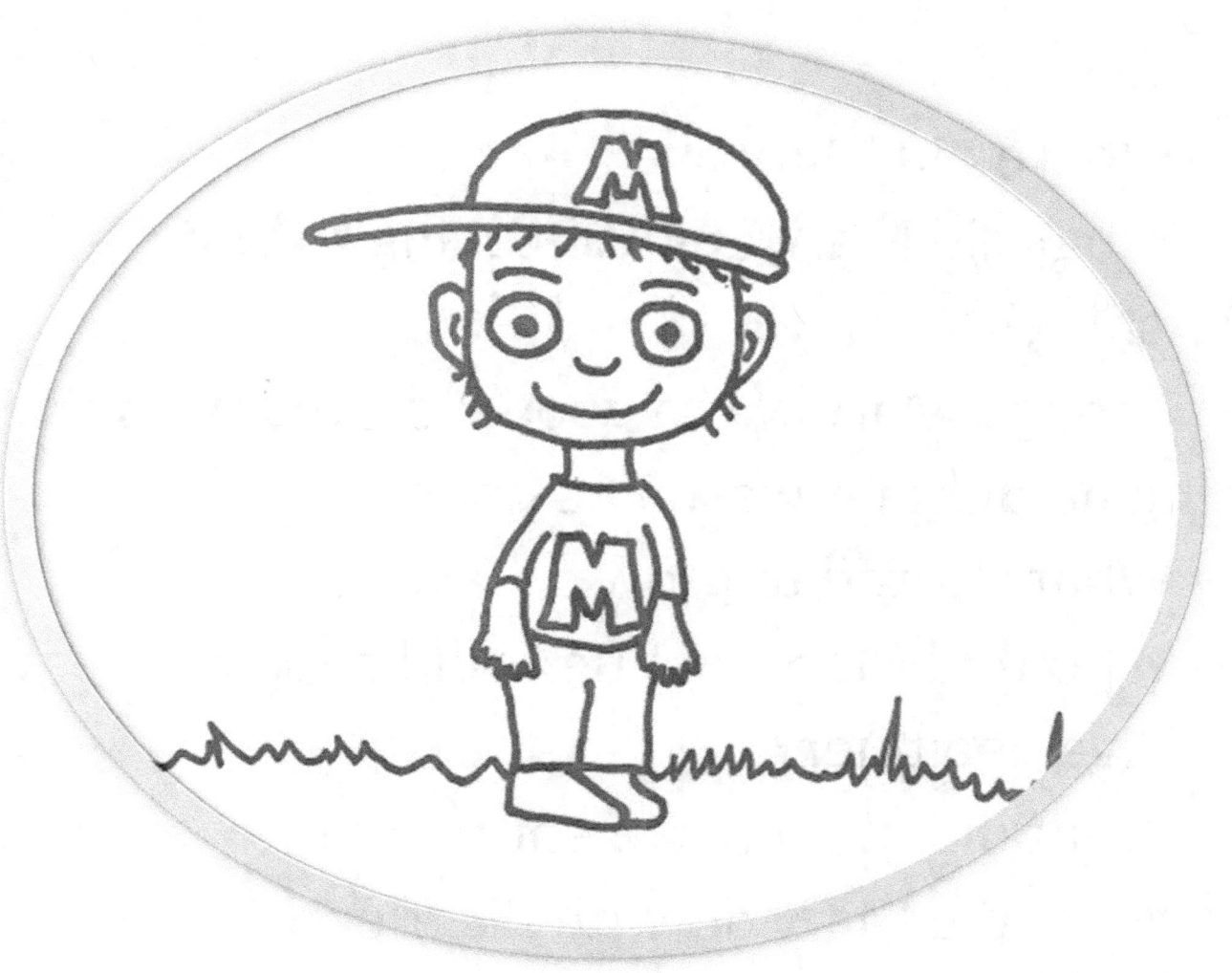

The End

Can you answer?

1.   Where did Marv live?
2.   What did Marv enjoy listening to and watching?
3.   Though Marv was a good kid, what was one thing he did that wasn't so good?
4.   What started to grow on Marv?
5.   Who told Marv that he could choose to eat and live healthier?
6.   What did Marv try to eat more of?
7.   What did Marv do with his friends?
8.   Can you start living healthier today?
9.   What are some things you like to eat?
10.   If someone tells you that you can't do better what can you tell them?

Marv's Healthy Choice

See how many words from this story you can find!

```
O N S I C D T R N N T H I L E E E N L I B E N R S
M B N K A A I G E F A N A W I C R L W H I J S O A
I E W G K V C I S A K Y O N G O S S E N A G K L S
I G O G K S A H T F I I B R W I D A K G L S H F F
N N R I Y C R J G G T C G G E V L A N C O U O I I
I F I H T T R N A Y H S E E E T D C I T A V A D S
O H G G I S I H G I A E K H E A K D V C N M D L
S G G U L K I T C E A K M Y G T O F C I I M S O O
I M R N L G M A A O G A S E O N N V A A O N Y A M
I F I A H I U M S G R N M G S A R K G D E N C N I
F O W L A W G L L V R E A R O M E I I L E I T K L
C O E K E K A S G E O C N A S I H A M G D A A S G
D H J D N G W F V K A S A C I T Y K I K V L S A D
F O I O C F E D F V E L H I N C I G I L A N E A L
R A S A G E B L I A L O Y A S I S N E S F A T B I
M G T K C G L T C N I N I E D L G E L I T S L L D
M I C E N L I I I C A N L A L I A I I A H G T I M
E L C L A I N E N R B D S T C O L A K M A C I E
I W N T N O O U G O A E V N J S M O O L O M K T I
T A A R H F F O F T C N L O G O R S N S I O S E S
A E T L I I E I E S I R T F C O R O S G A O C H A
K M E B O L L G L E L A O O G E S L O A D K S G I
C E L S W A E M T L A O D A G R I C N L I A O H K
N L L I C V Y R A L O L I F B G I M M M L S H K D
```

Marv	California	Food	Mom
Dad	Healthy	Snacks	Cookies
Smile	Talking	Walking	Jogging
Fruit	Vegetables	Choice	